ECCENTRIC DOCTORS

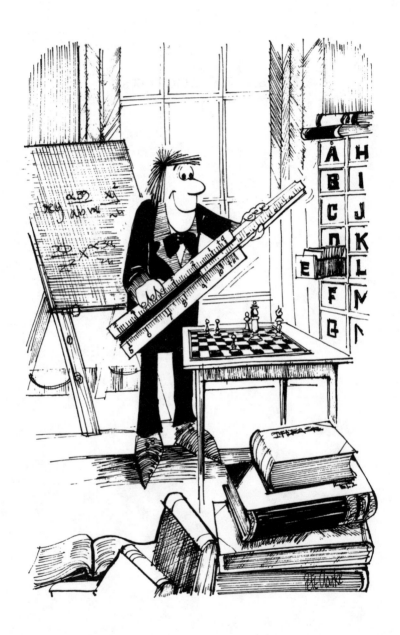

MOWBRAYS ECCENTRICS SERIES
Series Editor: J. A. Maxtone Graham

ECCENTRIC DOCTORS

by

ALAN WYKES

MOWBRAYS

LONDON & OXFORD

© A. R. Mowbray & Co Limited 1975

Photoset, printed and bound
in Great Britain by
REDWOOD BURN LIMITED
Trowbridge & Esher

ISBN 0 264 66173 7

First published in 1975 by A. R. Mowbray & Co Limited,
The Alden Press, Osney Mead, Oxford, OX2 0EG

Contents

INTRODUCTION   *Page* 7

1   William Price: 'This way to the Crematorium'   9

2   Sir Archibald McIndoe, c.b.e.: 'Put on your heaviest
    boots.'   14

3   John Hunter: Apoplectic anatomist   19

4   François Rabelais: Best-selling bawd   25

5   Simon Forman: Quackery, lechery, and magic   31

6   Anton Chekhov: Doctor without patients   36

7   Francis Galton: Disposal of the unfittest   41

8   Gerolamo Cardano: Odds and universal joints   47

9   Theodore Morell: The Führer's tricycling quack   53

10 Peter Roget: Snap! crackle!! pop!!!   58

Introduction

'A FUNNY lot, doctors', one of them once said to me. 'Can't even cure themselves as St Luke told them to.' (It wasn't St Luke: it was St Luke quoting Jesus, who was quoting a proverb; but never mind.) Well, they may be oddballs; but by and large it can't be claimed for them or charged against them that they are odder balls than the professionals in other fields. Nor can it be claimed that the collection presented here are the most or least famous or the oddest of them all. But they're my ten, chosen from a range that spans much of medical history. Some I had to leave out. St Luke himself was a physician, but odder as a writer than as a doctor, so biblical scholars tell us. Aesculapius, who gave the medical profession its symbol of a snake-entwined staff, was a sort of mythical Freud; John of Gaddesden, who featured as Chaucer's 'Docteur of Phisik', was also a doctor of souls in the guise of Canon of St Paul's cathedral and physician to the royals of his day, besides being the first recorded English gourmet; and David Livingstone is perhaps the most widely known of all because of his rescuer's famous greeting. But those displayed here seem to me to have combined their oddities with genuine contributions to the benefit and wealth of mankind. Not to mention mankind's health, which mankind has ever been concerned to set against the inevitability of death, as if death were some kind of pinnacle that could be conquered, like Everest.

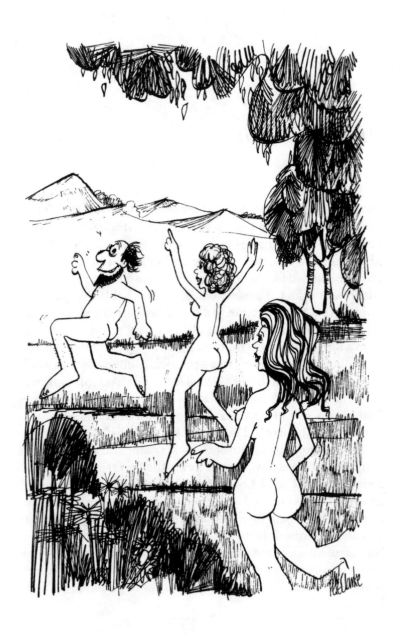

1 William Price: 'this way to the crematorium'

A CENTURY ago, in 1874, the Cremation Society was formed with the clearly stated object of 'disposing of the bodies of the naturally dead in a cleanly and solemn manner and without recourse to valuable ground space.' The founders of the Society were unknown loners, thought by the few who had heard of their dreadful idea to be dotty pyromaniacs, probably seeking a way of hiding the evidence of murder. That is, until the trial of Dr William Price.

Price lived and practised in Llantrisant, Glamorgan. His cures were often unconventional but invariably effective. At the time of his trial in 1884 he was eighty-four years old. His numerous children (he was to sire three more before he died) were all bastards, since he disapproved of marriage, which in his view chained women to their masters like slaves.

Besides being an unbeliever in marriage he was a vegetarian, a fanatical opponent of vaccination and tobacco, an ardent sun-worshipper and nudist who roamed his native Welsh hills and woods with an equally ardent bevy of young naked girls in his wake, a Chartist, and the self-appointed Archdruid of Wales. He believed in reincarnation, and when Helena Blavatsky founded the Theosophical Society in 1875 wrote to her claiming to be her father in a previous existence 10,000 years earlier. Blavatsky admitted the logic of this and enrolled him in the Society without fee.

The trial was at Cardiff Assizes before Mr Justice Stephenson. The charges were, first, attempting to obstruct the course of an inquest by burning a body and, secondly, attempting to dispose of a body by burning when the law required that it should be buried in hallowed ground. The Cremation Society, which in ten years had failed to establish the legality of its aims, sent an eagerly interested representative, Mr Joseph Glover, to hear William Price defend himself.

Defend himself he certainly did. He was what is known in the legal profession as 'a contentious litigant'. He would be in and out of the courts for the joy of argument – at which he was extremely good. But there was very little argument about the first of the charges against him. He triumphantly flourished the coroner's certificate proving that there had already been an inquest on the body in question – it was that of his infant son, whom he'd called, with typical disregard for convention, Jesus Christ – and death had been attributed to natural causes. Collapse of the Crown case.

As for the second charge, he challenged judge and jury to bring to light the legislation that made the burning of a dead body illegal.

At this stage the Minister of the church at Llantrisant was called upon as a witness and testified that the Church required that the body of any baptised infant be committed to hallowed ground.

'The Church is not the law', Price said. He raised his right hand, an impressive bearded figure dressed in a white robe embroidered with cabalistic signs, and continued a long and incomprehensible tirade in a gibberish that he claimed to be the ancient tongue of the Welsh bards. The judge, understandably, threatened him with an additional charge of contempt and had him taken from the court to cool down. When brought back to face the court again he told the judge naïvely that he had had no wish to offend but that he, the judge, was really the one at fault because he, Dr William Price, had been appointed by God the all-powerful among the Druids and was therefore superior in authority to anyone belonging to the mere Christian Church – a much newer institution in the scheme of things.

'Nevertheless', the judge said with considerable patience and self control, 'you will accept my authority in this court or go to gaol.'

There came now a chain of witnesses to testify both to his mad behaviour and to his prowess as a doctor. Of the former there were tales enough to raise the hair of the most impassive: tales of slavering dogs guarding his house, of blunderbusses used by his manservant and his housekeeper (who was also the mother of several of his children) when his privacy was threatened, of grave-robbery and the dissection of corpses. Many of them were doubtless trimmed with the poetic imagination of the Welsh; but they created an eerie sensation, and the reporters in the press benches could scarcely fashion their telling phrases fast enough.

Price, who had now shed his Druidical robe and sat resplendent in red and green coat, trousers and waistcoat, listened with amused attention 'as if', one reporter wrote, 'he was hearing of the deeds of someone other than himself.'

He took much more notice when witnesses – both patients and medical authorities – vouched for his skill as a doctor. His training had been authentic and he had taken his degree at the Royal College of Surgeons in 1821, returning to Wales to practise among those who needed him most and whom he understood best. The people of Llantrisant had a love-hate relationship with him: they were quick enough in their calls upon his treatments, but his oddities alarmed and angered them. However, they were generous in their acknowledgement of his understanding of their ways and ills.

One Huw Evans testified that Dr Price had cured him of 'consumption' (he hadn't tumbled to the fact that the consumption Price had cured him of was over-eating) by giving him a draught that was 'so bitter it kept me abed for weeks, look, with nothing to my insides but a gruel that could allay its foulness.' Several women said he was 'as gentle as a bird' (or words to that effect) at their confinements. And one miner spoke glowingly of the anaesthetic properties of the brandy Dr Price had administered prior to a leg amputation after a pit disaster. 'He would always come willing' was a phrase heard several times; 'he knew who could pay and who not' was another.

One way and another Price emerged from the witnesses' testimony rather more sinned against than sinning. Judge Stephenson took a long time over his summing up, first bringing the jury's thoughts back to the point at issue: that Dr Price was charged with burning the body of his own infant son, rather than burying it in the accepted manner, because, as the jury had heard, he was of the opinion that cremation was more wholesome than interment, and that the ancient religion to which Dr Price claimed to belong demanded the reduction of a corpse to ashes. In England 'in these enlightened times' every man was entitled to his own beliefs, and to follow the practices of religions more ancient than Christianity was not an offence in itself. However, it became an offence if it transgressed the laws of the land and of the present day. There was, the learned judge continued, no law except the law of custom and convention that precluded the burning of the corpses of those who had come to their end by natural causes, unless – and here the judge leaned forward to stress his point – unless the burning constituted a public nuisance. That was what the jury had to decide.

And that was what the jury could not decide. After a long absence the foreman reported that they could not agree: the evidence was too conflicting. There would have to be a new trial. Mr Joseph Glover telegraphed Sir Henry Thompson, the Cremation Society's founder, that they were still no nearer establishing the legality of the Society's object.

Then came a sensational development: the police decided not to proceed with the charge and Judge Stephenson, no doubt with considerable relief, recalled the jury and ordered it to discharge the doctor. Contentious litigant that he was, he at once brought charges against the police for malicious prosecution, defamation of character, and wrongful imprisonment. When the case came to court six months later the jury announced the verdict in his favour, but signified their contempt by limiting his damages to a farthing.

Even now that the legality of cremation had been established there remained considerable difficulties to be overcome by the Cremation Society. They were in continual conflict with the Home Office, whose advanced state of hydra-headedness produced delays and ambiguities for several years. The famous crematorium at Woking, 'specially constructed with regenerative and reverberating furnaces according to the Italian models' (it was the Italian chemists Polli and Brunetti who had worked out the speediest method of resolving corpses into gases), had very little reverberating or regenerating to do until 1902. In that year, eighteen years after the Price trial, the Act to legalise and regulate crematoria was passed.

Dr Price had of course determined his own method of being cremated: no built-in furnaces for him. He ordered that his corpse should be burnt publicly on Caerlan hill, sitting in an ancient chair on top of two tons of coal like a Guy Fawkes effigy. But that was in 1893 and the Home Office was only half way through its prevarications and ambiguities. Permission for such a hellish spectacle was refused. The corpse must be decently shrouded in a coffin first. The 20,000 spectators who paid threepence each to watch seemed not to mind. Glee and sorrow seemed to be about equally distributed among them: the love-hate relationship had not evened out with his death. Nobody from the Cremation Society was among the spectators – not officially anyway. But Sir Henry Thompson remarked on seeing the report in the *Glamorgan Echo*:

'A remarkable man.'

2 Sir Archibald McIndoe, C.B.E. 'Put on your heaviest boots'

ON THE EVENING of Saturday 18 April 1959.an extraordinary company of men assembled at number one Carlton House Terrace, once the London residence of that Very Superior Person Lord Curzon.

The men were all invalided air crews of the Royal Air Force. They had been horribly mutilated in battle and subsequently miraculously repaired, so that although their mutilations were still evident in scars, blindness, and the graftings of plastic surgery, they lacked nothing of the dignity, or the laughter and conversation, of whole men. They were the guests of the Savage Club – an assembly of men extraordinary in other ways – and their host for the evening was an Honorary Member of that club, Sir Archibald McIndoe, the restorer of their mutilations and at that time a man of world-wide fame for his skill, his egotism, and his unrelenting aggressiveness.

'I am well aware', he once told a newspaper man, 'that many people find me unbearable; but *everybody* finds me impossible to ignore.'

It was true. Though not remarkably large physically he seemed to fill any room he was in – even this one, once Lord Curzon's viceregal salon. His eyes, behind top-rimmed spectacles, had a cold and clinical glint in them despite a carefully composed smile; his hands, which were broad and stubby, with nails and skin abrasively raw from incessant scrubbing-up, gave the lie to the novelist's notion that surgeons have long, delicate, sensitive fingers. At the long top table his sometime

14

patients – his Guinea Pigs, as they called themselves – flanked him like a guard of honour, their conspicuous injuries attracting little attention from the club diners because McIndoe himself had, as usual, drawn the the limelight to himself.

'I know myself to be superior to any Very Superior Person who may once have occupied this room, he said, with a pretence of self-mockery in his after-dinner speech, 'because I am a renovator of men's faces – a face-lifter if you like – a restorer of confidence; and in a sense a spiritual healer. Thus I take to myself godlike status.'

The line got a laugh; and an even bigger laugh followed the extremely audible comment of an eminent Professor of Physics across the table from the speaker:

'The man's giving himself a remarkably good character.'

The comment was justified within the purlieus of that club, since it is unwritten Savage Club law that one's fame or achievements are discarded on entry – or, as the law is expressed, 'haloes are to be left in the hall.' But it might never have been made so far as McIndoe was concerned. He snapped off the laughter it gained in three seconds flat and continued with his speech, in which he told something of his life story.

He was a New Zealander, born in Dunedin in 1900, and educated at Otago High School. 'I passed *Medicinae et Chirurgiae Baccalaureus*, which is a posh way of saying Bachelor of Medicine and Surgery, when I was twenty-four; and the next six years opening people's abdomens in the Mayo Clinic, Rochester, Minnesota.'

His brilliance there was noted by the founders of the clinic, the brothers Mayo, who referred to him as 'the magician of the abdominal knife'. They also noted that his chin was that of 'a thruster – he'll never be backward in coming forward.'

Nor was he. He left the United States for London in 1930, more or less banking on a senior appointment in one of the leading hospitals. But this was the time of the depression and there were no appointments; no one seemed interested in him except his cousin, Sir Harold Gillies, a cosmetic surgeon of considerable eminence, who promised to 'drop a word or two where it might be useful' but urged him to make his own way as far as possible.

'It was then that I adopted an axiom: put on your heaviest boots and tread on anyone who gets in the way.'

He did just that – footing it rough-shod over colleagues, opponents, administrators and Governors alike; sometimes subtly, sometimes by blatant breaches of etiquette – 'An etiquette that works well for the lily-livered but never got anybody anywhere, so to hell with etiquette when I'm on my way up.'

He gained his Fellowship of the Royal College of Surgeons in 1932 and blazed his way to the job of General Surgeon at the Hospital for Tropical Diseases. Cousin Harold, who'd had some hand in the blazing, helped him further by shedding some of his private patients on to McIndoe, who was showing immense skill and interest in plastic surgery and in gaining insight into the 'sad psychology of rich people who wanted their dewlaps tightening up to convince themselves and others that they weren't so old as they appeared to be, or who had become cringing introverts because of facial blemishes or distortions.'

Since it was essential to him in his onward and upward march, he contrived a bedside manner. The façade of smiling welcome was created; and, being essential for his purpose, it stayed. The seven years of his life from 1932 to 1939, he later told his wife, were those in which he learnt compassion and a degree of understanding of the wretchedness of the ugly and misshapen.

It made him no less bullying in his manner, however, nor any less determined to remain in the limelight. The bulldozing methods had to stay. But there came a time when only a man with those methods could have succeeded in making a success of the job for which he was destined and into which he forced his way over the heads of three bitterly resentful rivals – the appointment of consultant to the Royal Air Force. All three of them, though, eventually and ungrudgingly admitted that, if ever the right man was in the right job, that man was McIndoe.

The appointment came in the summer of 1939, when war was inevitable; and McIndoe's first contemptuous assault was on the authorities 'who hadn't got around to realizing that there was no hospital that specialised in the repair work that the mutilations of battle would make necessary.'

The small Queen Victoria Hospital at East Grinstead in Sussex was in his opinion as near the ideal hospital as could be made without building from scratch ('Which there wasn't time for'). He set about adapting it with furious onslaughts on everything and everybody standing in the way. He terrified the Governors into submission to all his demands for extensions, alterations and installations by threatening the direst penalties for non-co-operation; equally, he bypassed all the proper Whitehall and Westminster channels in his determination to get materials and staff. When, after the blitz, a Minister refused to release building materials on the ground that he had 250,000 homeless to consider first, McIndoe got an audience with the King and the decision was reversed.

The earliest casualties of the Battle of Britain were the Guinea Pigs on whom he tried out new techniques for the grafting of bone, cartilage and fat, and the rehabilitation of limbs that might otherwise have become cripplingly deformed. They formed McIndoe's 'Guinea Pigs' Club' after the war and one of them wrote in the Club's journal of the 'marvellous psychological effect' brought by McIndoe's reassurances:

'He never claimed we'd resume the faces we were used to in the shaving mirror; but he chivvied us into a state of indifference to the sometimes horrified glances of the public, and into gradually losing our self-consciousness. That was a form of bullying too; but you knew at once it was the only way, that a more sentimental form of sympathy would simply have led to wallowing in self-pity. "Don't kid yourself you were ever beautiful," he used to say; "and you're going to be even less beautiful now. But you're going to get used to it, and everybody else is too. People are permanently concerned about their own affairs; only momentarily about yours. The world doesn't care, in the long term, what you or anybody else looks like. A child may say, 'Why is your face like that?' and you tell him and he accepts it and returns to his own affairs. Your contemporaries won't have to be told: they know. They'll feel a brief gratitude that it wasn't them and forget it. Match your indifference to theirs and you'll be all right.'''

It wasn't entirely true, but the reassurance was psychologically right. In any case, many of them were repaired with scarcely a blemish to be seen; but those invited to Carlton House Terrace that night were some of the worst cases – and some of the most enthusiastic about McIndoe's skill and character. 'He may have trampled on other people's feelings, but never on ours.'

3 John Hunter
apoplectic anatomist

HENRY FOX, statesman in Walpole's government and father of the more famous Charles James, wrote to his son at Eton in 1765: 'I am much put out by the building of a house, not so far from here as to quench alarm, wherein a magical chirurgeon lives who has dead bodies brought to him in carts and sustains wild animals whose crys and roars are to be heard often. It is said that even highway robbers dare not venture that far into the country.'

'The country' was the district of London now known as Earl's Court, and Fox was writing from Holland House, a residence he was later to own. The 'wild animals' were a few species of monkeys, some wild goats, a wolf or two, and a civet. To Fox, 'magical' meant mad; and the 'magical chirurgeon' was John Hunter, anatomist and surgeon of renown in the medical world, whose curiosity about the construction of human and animal bodies was boundless, and who had already, at the age of thirty-seven, advanced the theories and principles of anatomy so far that one of his fellow surgeons at St George's Hospital referred to his experiments as 'going beyond the bounds of lawful knowledge'. Hunter, always an irascible man, had justifiably replied that 'knowledge can only be increased by going outside its present bounds, and who believes that not to be so is a fool.'

It was true that cadavers were taken to him at Earl's Court. It was easy enough to buy them from impoverished relatives of the dead who cared more for money than for a respectable

19

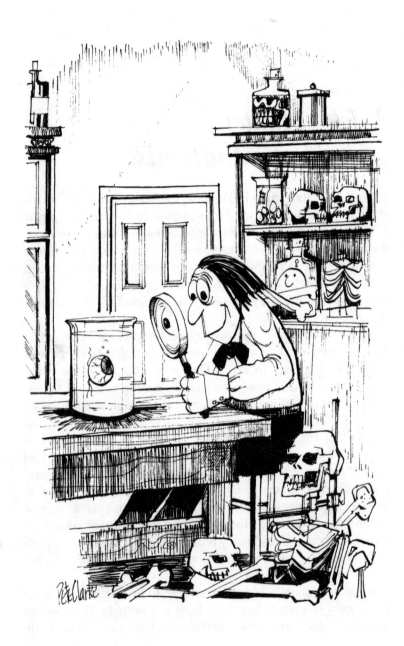

Christian burial. 'Will people rather have me cut up their bodies alive?' he testily asked his older brother William (also a surgeon and anatomist), 'that I may train my hands in discovering misteries?'

His manual dexterity had been acquired during his youthful apprenticeship as a cabinet-maker in Glasgow; his interest in animal life during his country childhood in Lanarkshire. William wrote of him that at fourteen he 'had much animal physiology in him from observing, from a lair in the woods, the habits of bees and small animals, and of setting them into captivity and dissecting them after their demise.'

He had little formal education and applied himself to reading and writing only because they could advance his exclusive concern with living things. His interest in games with other children was limited to the minor injuries they sustained when falling down, which he would dress and examine with all the application of a practised doctor. On one occasion, some small playmate having fallen from a swing, he assured the summoned physician that the injury was 'to the *tendo Achillis*' – a diagnosis that proved entirely accurate. He surprised the doctor further by suggesting the proper treatment of cold compresses and rest for twenty-four hours – 'after which as much circular movement of the limb should be encouraged to restore the running of the blood.'

When he was twenty, Hunter left Glasgow and travelled to London, arriving at his brother's house 'with an advanced anatomical knowledge of the horse deduced from his observations of the animal's movements observed during the journey.' His pockets were full of scraps of paper on which he had been drawing diagrams of the animal's muscles as he supposed them to lie under the flesh – 'not accurate, but not so very wrong either.'

As his brother's assistant and pupil he had every opportunity of watching innumerable obstetrical operations, for William was surgeon-accoucheur at the Middlesex Hospital. The pupil took a gruesome interest in collecting and preserving specimens that were, so to speak, the throwaways from the operating tables: teeth, splinters of bone from gunshot wounds, aborted

foetuses, fingernails, bits of cranium and vertebrae, and pre-
served organs of human and animal bodies, all found their way
into his rooms in Soho where he examined them minutely and
built up a display for his own pupils to learn from. (He collected
over 10,000 in his lifetime and they eventually became the prop-
erty of the Royal College of Surgeons and the mainstay of the
Hunterian Museum; but much of the collection was destroyed
by enemy action in 1941.)

His skills were much more widely spread than those of the
modern surgeon, who invariably specialises. Hunter was a bio-
logist, a physiologist, a pathologist, a botanist, a haemotologist,
and a venereologist – not to mention a General Practitioner of
extreme competence. His promised appointment as Sur-
geon-Extraordinary to George III enabled him to persuade the
Admiralty to let him go as a ship's surgeon during the naval
attack on the French possession Belle-Île-en-Mer in 1760 'so
that he could be among the wounded and dying, save those it
was possible to save by surgery, and dissect the bodies of those
that succumbed.'

From Belle-Île he went on to serve with the British military
forces in Portugal, who were busily engaged in evicting the
Spaniards from Lisbon, and in the intervals between stitching
up the living and dissecting the dead made a collection of hundreds of animals which he took back with him to England and
installed in the house in Golden Square where in 1773 he set up
in private practice.

Since he did much of his dissecting work at night in a ground-
floor uncurtained room facing on to the square, his bloody activities aroused considerable alarm; and it was for that reason
that he transferred his activities to Earl's Court, where his isola-
tion was assured because few had the courage to go near the
'magical chirurgeon' in case they should fall victim to his dissecting knife.

Unfortunately he was himself a victim – not of the knife but of
angina pectoris, that heart condition characterised by brief
spasms of extreme pain that can be caused by any unwonted activity or raising of the blood pressure. 'My life', he wrote to

brother William, 'is in the hands of any rascal who chooses to annoy and tease me.' But his life was very much in his own hands too; and in his determination to prove that the diseases of gonorrhoea and syphilis were the same he deliberately infected himself with the syphilitic bug *spirochaeta pallida*. It was one of the occasions when he was wrong: they are quite different organisms. He was to pay for his error. Though he never reached the paralytic or organic disruption that, for example, overtook Hitler, there can be no doubt that the self-inflicted disease lessened the resistance power of his already stammering heart.

However, he allowed nothing to interfere with the course of his work, which included the preparation and delivery of nearly a hundred lectures to students on the theory and practice of surgery. At all of these, surreptitious warnings were passed round before the start not to put questions that might arouse Hunter's contempt or indignation. He was always to be cherished rather than challenged.

To be sure, few of his pupils had the knowledge or the wit to challenge him: such challenges came, if at all, from his contemporaries. They tended to reproach him as scientists are reproached today for venturing into fields unknown. To press 'beyond the bounds of lawful knowledge' was a suspect and in some ways sacrilegious activity, and Hunter's treatises and lectures investigated anatomical concepts very different from those so far understood. But they usually proved to be right. For example, the modern treatment of the common thrombosis in the area behind the knee derives entirely from Hunter's experiments on deer, when he severed the main artery to the antler and proved that the circulation can be restored by binding up the affected conduit and allowing nature to take its course. Nothing so revolutionary had been heard of in days when amputation was the standard answer to such problems.

Gradually, however, his theories became accepted. William Heberden, Dr Johnson's physician and one of his firmest supporters, sponsored him for Fellowship of the Royal Society, and introduced him to the girl who became his wife – Anne Home, a

pop-song writer of the day who wrote the words of several dit-
ties that were set to music by Haydn, including *My Mother Bids
me Bind my Hair*. Anne was the ideal wife for Hunter: she had a
calming effect on him, persuaded him to rest frequently, and
kept herself in the background. She was literally in the background of the portrait Reynolds painted of Hunter (now in the
Royal College of Surgeons) but asked the artist to efface her
'because my life is one of triviality compared with the Parnassus
from which my husband addresses the world.'

It was a considerably smaller gathering he was addressing
from the eminence of his Parnassus on 16 October 1793: speci-
fically the Board of Governors of St George's Hospital, his
Alma Mater. One of them was suddenly misguided enough to
challenge him on his opinion of the causes of George III's
increasingly frequent attacks of insanity, which Hunter main-
tained were genetic factors. (He was right, as subsequent researches have proved.) Hunter was so furious at his challenger's
stupidity that he had an apoplectic seizure and collapsed across
the board-room table, to die within a few minutes. He was
sixty-five.

Hunter's researches and behaviour had been accounted so
odd by government bureaucrats – spurred on by Henry Fox –
that official disapproval disdained his magnificent museum of
specimens for six years after his death. Only in 1799 was the
collection bought, grudgingly, for £15,000 (it had cost Hunter
in his lifetime more than £75,000) and given into the care of the
Royal College of Surgeons. And another sixty years passed
before his mortal remains were given a place of honour in Westminster Abbey – to which they were translated from St Martin-
in-the-Fields. By that time he had been acknowledged as the
instigator of truly scientific surgery. Before him, practically all
surgery was hit-and-miss; after him – well, one might say that
he gave his heart to Christian Barnard.

4 *François Rabelais* *best-selling bawd*

Monseigneur Jean du Bellay, Bishop of Paris, was on his way to Rome to receive his Cardinal's hat in October 1533 when terrible pains in his hips and buttocks forced him to stop at Lyons. He was virtually unable to move and had to be carried, shouting far from holy oaths, from his coach to the nearest inn. The innkeeper, impressed by the status of his improbable visitor, sent a message urgently to the local teaching hospital, the Hôtel-Dieu. Could any physician be spared to attend to Monseigneur in his agony?

In response to this *cri de coeur* came a youthfully middle-aged man wearing a fur-edged robe and a skull cap decorated with a golden scarab, and having a merry face adorned with a clipped beard. This was François Rabelais, lecturer in anatomy at the hospital. He was thought by his colleagues of the medical fraternity to be dangerously mad because of his many clashes with the Church and the philosophers. The Renaissance was not a good time to conflict with established opinion on any fundamental matter.

Rabelais, however, argued with priests about the validity of their spiritual cures, with doctors and apothecaries about their physicks, and with patients about the extent of their illnesses.

Monseigneur's pains he quickly diagnosed as sciatica, applied some balm which he promised would give some temporary relief, and demanded ten gold louis.

The Bishop almost fainted with another kind of pain – the threat to his purse. 'But that's a fortune! And quite unjustified

25

by the brevity of your visit and the amount of attention you've given me!'

'One louis', Rabelais replied scathingly, 'for the time and the balm; nine for being able to tell you the nature of your illness' – and thereby became the coiner of the apothegm.

He was no respecter of persons, or of ideas in opposition to his own straightforward rationalism. The son of a lawyer, he was born in the early part of the last decade of the fifteenth century at Chinon in the Loire valley. He had been a monk of both open and closed orders (he found the Franciscans intent on 'nothing but the good death') and was openly lustful in an age when much lust was hidden behind a façade of sobriety.

'Original sin and the fall of man', he claimed, 'is a doctrine manifested by woe and hand-wringing.'

As a young man he had attacked the crying abuses of the Church, the monasteries that had become the refuge of the worthless and lazy, and all those who placed stumbling blocks in the paths of seekers after true learning. His attacks were couched in such boisterous terms that he escaped arrest and punishment because it was assumed that no one who would take such risks could be mentally normal.

Guarded by such welcome dismissal he studied botany, architecture, law, and education, and wrote treatises on all these subjects in terms of such literary buffoonery that could only confirm the opinions of others of his mental instability.

Despite his supposed dottiness he entered the profession of medicine at Montpellier – the leading French medical Faculty of the time – and matriculated as a Bachelor of Medicine in 1530. He could not afford to stay on and work for his Licentiate, having spent all his income on carnal pleasures; so he left shortly after qualifying and decided to become a best-selling writer.

Unlike many of those who attempt the same thing today, he had the talent; also the perspicacity to settle for stories that the public wanted. Popular success lay in the churning out of innumerable romances and allegories. (Boccaccio's *Decameron* had set the fashion more than a century previously). He quickly seized on a folk tale of the period about a giant called Gargantua, elaborated it in an acceptable manner by extending Gargantua's adventures to those of an invented son, Pantagruel, and publishing it under the portentous title *Les Horribles et espouvantables faictz et prouesses du très renommé Pantagruel, Roy de Dipsodes, fils du grant géant Gargantua.*

The dreadful deeds of Pantagruel were denounced with the greatest vehemence by the syndics of the Sorbonne and pronounced forbidden reading by Pope Clement VII. In consequence there was a great rush to buy the book by surreptitious means. (Those who risked excommunication by reading it had it bound to look like a holy book.) Everyone was enchanted by its merry coarseness (including, naturally, the syndics and the Pope). Its imaginative descriptions of the bodily functions, its learned but lighthearted references to all the parts of the body – with special emphasis, so to speak, on the genitalia – and its pointed satire on the establishment had all the makings of a best seller.

'Only a doctor could have written such a book,' the wiseacres rightly observed; and they determined – or made a show of determining – to cast him out from the profession. But not one of them spotted Monsieur le Docteur François Rabelais behind the anagrammatic pseudonym he had made of his name – Alcofribas Nasier. As Nasier he simply stood back and let the fortune from the sale of its numerous editions fall into his lap.

Also into his lap fell Roberte Vimeux, a pretty girl still in her teens who had been courted by a swineherd whom she treacherously cast aside for the favours of the newly rich author, who found her innocence engaging and 'too good not to pluck'. Their son Théodule died at the age of two; but according to a scurrilous letter sent to the Abbot of the Benedictine abbey of St-Maur-le-Fossé, his natural children were 'as the stars of heaven'.

The Abbot, who was at that time none other than Jean du Bellay, replied that the doings of an unidentifiable doctor, however reprehensible, were scarcely anything to do with him, but that machinery and funds existed for the care of fallen girls; also a convent into which they could be taken to make penance for their wicked acts.

It was at this stage that du Bellay came up for preferment and was laid low in Lyons on his way to Rome. He paid Rabelais his ten louis under strong protest, said that it was barbarous to blackmail a sick man and prophesied that the doctor, however healing his fingers, would find no joy in heaven.

'A fig for that,' Rabelais replied. 'All my joys are earthly ones. And my sorrows too, come to that – like yours. But I see a way of our helping each other. I will accompany you to Rome without further fee as your physician, easing your pains when they occur, if you will procure for me the pardon and release from the convent at St-Maur of a young woman too young and gay to be caged up with all those fluttering crows.'

The Bishop considered. It would certainly be an advantage to him to have a medical attendant; it would also add considerably to his prestige with his fellow clergy. . . .

'The woman's name?'

'Roberte Vimeux.'

'Ah! So you must be none other than – '

'Of course. It amused me to hide behind a façade as crumbling as that presented by those blindly orthodox scions of Church and out-dated philosophy. I intend to continue the attack with many more of the adventures of Gargantua and Pantagruel. It is only through the vast appetites of human nature for food and drink and laughter that any kind of humanity can be achieved.'

This cryptic remark unnerved the Bishop as much as the discomfort of his sciatica; but he struck the bargain and Rabelais accompanied him to Rome, Roberte having been settled comfortably in Montpellier. Here the unorthodox doctor returned and continued his medical studies until 1537, when he was granted his Licentiate. He also continued the production of the stories of Gargantua and Pantagruel, for which there was an ever-waiting audience. (Some 200 editions had been published by the end of the nineteenth century.) Through them he mocked medieval Catholicism and Calvinism, both of which adopted attitudes of dogmatic tyranny that made ignorance a virtue.

The extreme coarseness of his language and imagery could be compared with some of today's novels, although his benevolent giants are considerably more comic. His satire is always benign (unlike that of his later countryman Voltaire) and without a trace of the equivocal licentiousness and sniggering indecency of later times and writers. He was unorthodox enough not only to feel deeply and sincerely but to express in jest what he felt in earnest, deliberately adopting his farcical technique as the vehicle of his opinions on subjects which it was then extremely dangerous to discuss. His philosophy rests ultimately upon the then heretical belief in the absolute goodness of Nature and what is natural. Much of his teaching, of his ideas in education, of his inspired humour, and of his advocacy of disinterested work for the good of humanity, has as direct an application in the modern world as it had in sixteenth-century France. In his time he was as great, and as deviant, as the giants he created for his Utopian world.

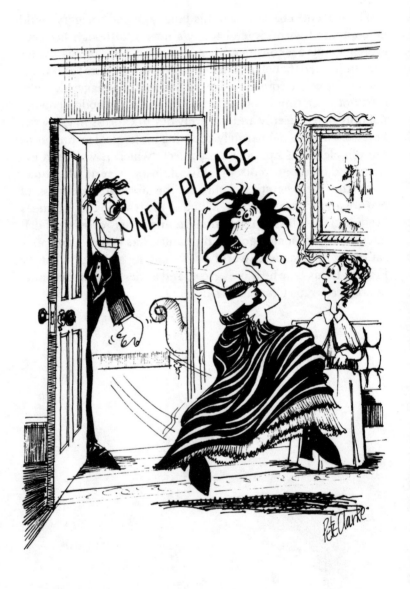

5 Simon Forman
quackery, lechery and magic

LIKE JOHN Wellington Wells in *The Sorcerer*, Simon Forman was a dealer in magic and spells. Also, he claimed, a doctor, though the Royal College of Physicians had dismissed him from their distinguished portals snarling 'mountebank' and 'charlatan'. Since he had never had any formal medical training, they had some justification. But Forman was indifferent. A continual stream of patients beat a path to his house in Lambeth for consultations.

For other things too, evidently. His diary for 9 July 1607 records: 'Halek 8 a.m. Hester Sharp, and halek at 3 p.m. Anne Wiseman, and halek at 9 p.m. Tronco.' Tronco was his wife, the others were ladies of little virtue and much lust. 'Halek' was his code word for coition. He was fifty-five in 1607: perhaps he was good at taking his own medicines. He compounded love philtres for the lovelorn, aphrodisiacs for the listless, and charms for the impotent; though judging by that busy day in 1607, no woman need have remained childless if a patient of 'Doctor' Forman. 'He bedded me,' one gullible lady wrote with astonishment, 'and there was no more to it than that. Now I am round with child, and it is his doing.'

Simon Forman's house in Lambeth had three consulting rooms. One was for those seeking medical treatment and analysis of character by means of metoposcopy – that is, the study of the features, especially the lines on the forehead and facial warts; a second was filled with the apparatus of astrology and the telling of fortunes; and the third was a kind of marriage

31

bureau in which he effected the assignations of those seeking
partners. The routine seems to have been for the hopeful pair to
be introduced and left to converse, thence to the astrological de-
partment for the casting of horoscopes to determine their suit-
ability, and finally to the surgery for the concoction of potions
to settle their course in life.

One of his best customers was Frances Howard, daughter of
Lord Howard of Bindon, who went to him first as a young girl
troubled with 'night flutterynges of the heart'. He told her, with
some logic, that she must come to him one night when her heart
was fluttering. This she did, and, she said, 'he devoided me of
my nyght-gowne and, having give me a potion to drive out
devills, soothed me uponn my breasts until I was plees'd.' Most
unethical. But she went again when she was older and asked
him to cast her life before her 'that I might see to what estate I
should be raysed.'

Forman sat her amid the clutter of astrolabes, globes, calen-
dars, charts, and almanacks, and cast her horoscope – 'his
beard brystlyng and his eye bryte.' (Nothing about wandering
hands, so presumably he behaved himself.) By her fortune, he
told her, she should 'change her estate' three times. She married, first, the son of a wealthy alderman of the city who 'dy'd
leaving me unchilded'; after his death she hooked an Earl, and
– he also leaving her widowed – finally nothing less than a
Duke. So in at least one proven case his fortune-telling proved
to be accurate. But as he was the recognised oracle of the day it
is reasonably certain that his prophesies were fulfilled frequently. Anxious merchants worrying about their argosies,
churchmen seeking preferment, lovers wanting to do away with
their rivals, gamblers urgently needing a change of fortune –
they all went to Simon Forman for reassurance.

Two of his best-known clients were Shakespeare's mistress
Emilia Lanier (she was also, most probably, the 'Dark Lady' of
the Sonnets) and his landlady, Mrs Mountjoy. Master Shakespeare, it appears, was behind with his rent and she sought to
know the likelihood of his future success, perhaps wondering
whether she should throw young Will into the street before her

losses became too big. History is voluble on the subject of his success but silent on whether Mrs Mountjoy rid herself of her troublesome tenant. But Forman gave her a posset 'to ease her humor' – by which he meant her state of health rather than her temper.

The necromantic side of Forman's practice was demonstrated most effectively on a rich merchant, Sir Barrington Molyns, who reported suffering from 'stinking sweet and venomous worms' in his nose. Forman told him demons had taken charge of him and must be cast out.

'I was given first a great purge of the herb Demonifuge,' Molyns records; 'then my flesh was pounded beneath stones which left no bruises but which, my benefactor said, were grinding the bones of the devil that lurked within me and if I would but listen I would hear the screams from the tortured thing. There was in truth a great ringing in my ears, so who is to say that it was not the sound of the demon within me being driven out? Nor was that all. Nearby was a pool of stagnant water, with toads leaping upon its edges, which were rich with slime. Here I had to go at midnight in the light of a full moon reflected in the pool, and immerse my head where the moon lay while all the vapours of the spell of which I was a victim were drawn upward to the atmosphere. After this I was to dry my head on unfouled straw from a nearby byre and reward my benefactor with a pouch of powdered alicorn,* which I did and completed my release from my bondage.'

A messy business necromancy, obviously, and well worthy of the frowns of the Royal College of Physicians; but they need not have hounded him so tenaciously. Like spies in a Watergate conspiracy they watched his house, sent phoney patients to bug his consultations, and organised posses of footpads to waylay him on dark nights and mutter threats as they held him against walls. According to Forman himself they did this 'hundreds of times'; but one must make allowances for his undoubted paranoia, which led him eventually to commit suicide.

Long before that, however, Cambridge University gave him a

* Powdered horn of the unicorn.

licence to practise 'the cure of ills of all kindes and substances of the human boddy.' With that authority he added many patients to his already thriving practice, accumulated a fortune in money and valuables (many of which he passed on to his enthusiastic partners in 'halek'), and built a new wing onto his house to accommodate bigger and better apparatus, stills, cauldrons, and the chests to hold his wealth and fine clothes. Tronco, his wife, enjoyed her husband's new prosperity – and apparently raised no objections to his extramarital 'halek'.

Despite his predeliction for the mystical and alchemical, Forman seems to have cured his patients of a great many ordinary ailments by quite ordinary means. His numerous casebooks indicate that in a single year (1604) he had over 500 successes – most of them, no doubt, with cut fingers, tooth extractions, wart removals, 'coffs & chokyngs', simple limb fractures, and the everyday transactions of a busy doctor's consulting room. The great cure-all of the day was bleeding, by leeches or other means; the theory being that only by the draining off of the infected blood could the patient be restored. But Forman rarely practised bleeding. The remedies noted in his prescription book and treatment book are usually less harsh: euphorbium for palsy, turpeth (mercuric oxysulphate) for croup, diarob (double strength grape juice) as a vehicle for carrying the more unpleasant emetics, white arsenic for lipyria, snake venom for 'dropsicall afflictions'. The syndics of Cambridge University sagely inspected his books before granting him their certificate and must have been satisfied that, if he killed some patients, he at least didn't kill more than other doctors despatched by their bleeding.

The Royal College of Physicians, however, continued to hound him with their spies, many of whom worked protection rackets of their own and took his money for the favour of reporting that they had found nothing untoward going on. With or without bribes such reports could have been nothing but a fair distance from the truth. What with his insemination of ladies with impotent husbands, his frivols with other ladies less embarrassed, his intrigues with ladies and gentlemen of the upper crust, his dealings with toads in slimy ponds, his braziers and alleged compacts with the devil, there can scarcely have been any moment of any day when something untoward wasn't going on. Either his rich full life or his paranoia did for him in the end, and he died from one of his own drafts on 11 September 1611. But a farcical version of his career was concocted by Ben Jonson in *The Alchemist*, and may be seen and read to this day.

6 Anton Chekhov
doctor without patients

Moscow University, 1884. A young man, very pale and thin, emerged from the Faculty of Medicine into the thin spring sunlight carrying a scroll of parchment.

'You must now heal the sick,' he had been told. 'According to the thirteenth volume of the Legal Code you may withhold your skill from no one. You must go always when called – whether it be aneurism or a toothache, and whether the caller be rich or poor. It is your duty to go.' The Principal had a narrow beard, divided into two spikes, very fierce. He drummed his fingers on his writing table. 'Your progress has been reasonable. Nothing astonishing, but you have worked hard. I have no doubt you will make a good provincial doctor.'

The young man was Anton Pavlovich Chekhov, third of the six children of Páviel Chekhov, the unsuccessful proprietor of a grocer's shop in Taganrog, a small town edging on the Azov Sea in south Russia. Páviel was a gifted amateur musician and painter but a rotten business man, always teetering on the brink of bankruptcy. Unstable in character, he hovered between the despotic, dealing out thrashings for trivial offences, and the grossly sentimental, smothering his children and his wife Yevghéniya with glutinous affection.

No one nowadays thinks of Chekhov as a doctor: he is Chekhov of *The Seagull*, and *The Cherry Orchard*, and *Three Sisters*, and the masterly short stories that, with de Maupassant's, have had what Somerset Maugham called 'the crowning influence' on English fiction of the twentieth century. But as he was to write

36

years later to his wife, the actress Olga Knipper, 'It was all there – the richness and poverty of life and humanity – in the sickrooms of my youth.'

No doubt. But what was conspicuously absent was the money to pay him with. His patients offered him hospitality – 'I could drown in the outpourings of their samovars' – and little else. He may have been legally subject to the demands of the rich, but it was always the poor who called him. The confinements of foundry workers' wives, the broken bones of farm workers tumbling from the tops of hayricks, the infections of children, the outbreaks of typhus in prison and workhouse – they brought a few roubles stretched over many months in pathetically small donations, but most of those roubles went to stop up the holes in the permanently leaking money bucket of feckless father Páviel. He was always ill-clothed against the bitter Russian winters, often undernourished, and much troubled with a weakness of the chest.

It was then that the young doctor had the Idea. In every sickroom he listened to meandering tales of family quarrels, of adulteries, of unwarranted poverty because of riches stolen or embezzled, of priests and rich merchants and musicians who never quite made it, of a child who became famous but forgot his parents in the grandeur of being appointed as engineer on the Trans-Siberian Railway. . . .

'I feel', he wrote, 'that it is not so much a doctor they need as a confidential receptacle into which they may pour their outbursts against supposed injustice, against life in general . . . they think me most peculiar, but they bargain with me and I with them. I make their miseries and joys into little stories, emphasizing or otherwise adjusting to give shape, and my friend Leykin buys them for his magazine *Splinters*; he always wants jokes and vignettes to fill holes in the paper and he's willing to pay . . . the money I put to the credit of my patients . . . so really I have no patients at all – only material.'

His by-line was The Doctor Without Patients, which took the fancy of many *Splinters* readers; but they mistook the intended irony for a plea and wrote that they would gladly become the sad doctor's patients . . . they had many unusual complaints and illnesses that they felt sure he would find interesting and would no doubt find recompense enough for his skill. . . .

He took on all he could, working sometimes seventeen hours a day, but using much of the time he spent at patients' houses making notes – which patients imagined to be prescriptions or reports to specialists at the hospital, or investigations into new and unknown diseases.

'People are not content with a simple hernia or a fracture of the finger; they turn everything into the rarest of diseases. It gives them immense satisfaction to think that their illnesses are different from everyone else's, that they are in some way unique because their grandfather or uncle was present during an outbreak of smallpox, and mixed smallpox with drink or a fall on the head, or because a drunken husband aimed a blow at someone's head, or because a child had a fright in the night.'

Transmuted by the story-teller's art, his bedside notes brought him an increasing reputation with editors, if not with patients. (To be sure, he was not all that good a doctor: his interests were philosophical rather than scientific.) Leykin published a collection of stories in volume form which attracted another editor, Souvorin of the St Petersburg daily *Novoye Vremya*. Souvorin immediately commissioned Chekhov to provide a second volume 'of longer and more serious tales – for I feel you have it in you to give us more substantial fare than we find in your little squibs and anecdotes.'

But his apparent indifference to the profits of medicine brought him into conflict with officialdom. The District Medical Superintendent, a pompous man who lived his life by rules and regulations, thought it extremely suspicious that Chekhov's ledgers should record so much in the wrong columns:

'There must be something amiss here' – the Superintendent stabbed with his pen at an entry – 'for you have *credited* the coachman Posrednik with forty roubles for the visits you made him during the year. This must be obscuring some defalcation.

The Legal Code, thirteenth volume, requires you to make a charge per visit. What are you covering up?'

'On the contrary,' Chekhov said, 'I am revealing rather than concealing, that although I could help myself to the bones my patients provide for my stories, my conscience does not allow me to do so. By crediting them with some of the money I'm paid by editors and publishers I leave them unruffled by the thought of debts they owe the doctor – and therefore easier to cure.'

'It's most irregular,' the Superintendent said. 'Very irregular indeed. I must make a report. I don't like it. I don't like it one little bit.'

Fortunately there were others who viewed Chekhov's indifference to rules and regulations with more tolerance. In 1892 he was himself appointed a District Medical Superintendent – 'Though I am aware that the appointment is more in acknowledgement of my literary stature than my medical efficiency, for I cannot even understand what is wrong with my own body. I cough, have palpitations, sometimes a haemorrhage. . . .'

He had been awarded the Pushkin prize by the Imperial Academy of Sciences and elected a member of the Society of Lovers of Russian Literature. His financial position had become secure, though much of his income still went to support his indolent family; and he was turning his attention to the theatre. But his health was failing alarmingly. And if he himself was unable to understand the cause, other doctors could. They diagnosed consumption and insisted that he must move to a warmer climate. Thereafter he became a much travelled man, but his search was always 'for life as lived by the people, the funny little people' rather than for restoration of his own health.

His fellow writers Tolstoi and Gorky found in him 'many peculiarities'. At a time when his chest was giving him considerable pain he insisted on carrying out a census of the convicts on Saghalien Island on the far side of Siberia – 'a journey that is madness in itself,' said Tolstoi; 'and for what purpose except to count criminals, the dregs of humanity?'

Chekhov saw things differently. There were no dregs of humanity: only people who were the victims of circumstance and of their own characters. In his plays, which deal with the decline of the Russian landed gentry, the characters take refuge in elaborate and impossible dreams of renewed prosperity. His stories never have plots in the accepted sense but delineate situations that arise from the nature of the people in them. D. H. Lawrence called him a 'Willy wet-leg' for his lack of robustness and scornfully added that 'He was an oddity of a doctor who has become an oddity of a writer – too odd to become of any importance.' An odd thing in itself for a writer of Lawrence's stature to say in 1928, by which time there was no possible doubt about Chekhov's importance.

Importance was something he never hankered after. He saw humanity as uniformly important, himself no more and no less than anyone else. He was disappointed when his plays failed – as *The Seagull* did at its first performance. (Two years later, in 1898, it was produced with such riotous success by the Moscow Arts Theatre that the company adopted a seagull as their emblem.) But there was no bitterness in him.

His travels to warmer places could not defeat the inroads made by tuberculosis and he died, aged forty-four, at the German health resort of Badenweiler, on 2 July 1904. Self-effacing to the last, he wrote to the Treasurer of the Mutual Aid Society of Doctors, who had asked for some details for the Faculty records:

'I suffer from a disease called autobiographphobia. To read any particulars about myself and, worse still, to write them down for publication is a real torment to me. But I have no doubt that the study of medicine has had an important influence on my literary work. It has considerably widened the range of my observation, and enriched me with knowledge, the value of which, to me, as a writer, can be understood only by one who is himself a doctor – albeit a very very odd one, as has been declared many times!'

7 Francis Galton
disposal of the unfittest

BURLINGTON HOUSE, November 1869. The Fellows of the Royal Society listened intently to the lecturer, Francis Galton, a broad man with a snood of white hair, bushy eyebrows, and thin lips. He was talking about the theory set forth in his newly published book *Hereditary Genius*, and they understood him to say that he advocated the 'suppression' of weak links in any hereditary human chain.

'Even by death?' asked one astonished Fellow.

'Certainly,' replied Galton, 'if necessary.' He emphasised that among animals runts did not survive.

Being scientists, they were unmoved by the social implications of exterminating unsatisfactory human strains. And Francis Galton was in no sense a man one could suspect of wicked intentions. A pillar of Victorian society, one might have called him. A Quaker of solid yeoman stock, his immediate ancestors were bankers, manufacturers, scientists in a small way. His cousin was the famous Charles Darwin, and his wife, Louisa Butler, came from a family with considerable distinction in the academic field. The family lived in Birmingham and he became a medical student at the city's General Hospital at the age of sixteen, transferring to King's College, London, a year later.

He displayed intense curiosity about the human body and the human mind. 'Admirable,' the Principal said, 'but not pointed in the proper direction. Mr Galton must keep to the curriculum. His present experiments will be the death not only

41

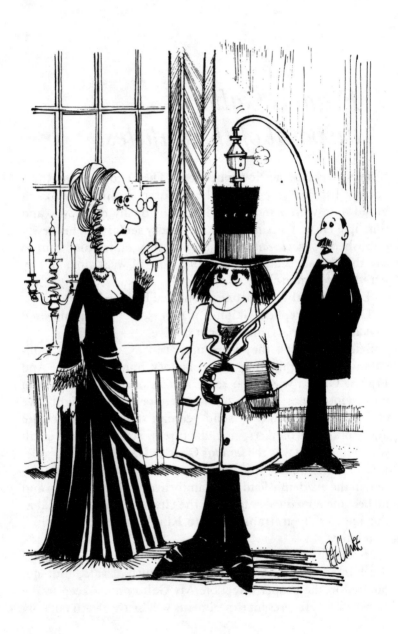

of himself but of his mentors also.'

Galton – he was seventeen at the time – had decided that the pharmacopoeia told him too little about the practical effects of products of the dispensary; he decided to sample everything himself, in strict alphabetical order. Aniseed and belladonna proved harmless, but the purgative effect of castor oil halted him at the third letter – 'Though not in my passage to the jakes, where I resolved that the method was too startling to the system.' Years later in his famous *Art of Travel* he advised those wishing to 'clear the system' to 'drink a charge of gunpowder in a tumblerful of warm water or soap-suds, and tickle the throat.' Clearly gunpowder has a less explosive effect when drunk than when fired.

At Trinity, Cambridge, to which Galton went at eighteen, he continued attending medical lectures. But his degree, when he took it, was in mathematics – which, he said, caused him to suffer a 'sprained brain'.

Sprained or not, his brain continued to expand its grip on countless subjects – all of them scientific. His father having left him a small fortune, he could have idled his days away in sybaritic luxury; but he chose to expand both his physical and mental capacities by travel, investigation of natural phenomena, and 'the advancement of racial perfection'. Like the doctors who preceded him by three centuries, he apparently believed that health was governed by 'humors', so he constantly wore a 'Patent Ventilating Hat', which allowed the supposedly overheated head to breathe by way of a valve controlled by a small bulb at the end of a rubber tube dangling from the crown. He always politely asked the hostesses of the dinner parties he attended for permission to wear this remarkable headgear 'in order not to embarrass your guests by falling in a fit upon the floor.' One might suppose from this that he had a Goonish sense of humour; but there is nothing in his written work to support the notion of humour of any kind.

Of all natural phenomena, Francis was specially interested in the weather. Espy's *The Philosophy of Storms* caused him, according to his soldier cousin Douglas, 'to become quite agitated with enthusiasm and to manipulate the shutters in his hat with remarkable rapidity.' His passionate belief in statistics enabled him to prepare weather charts of greater accuracy than had been known (the direct antecedents of those on today's television) and to establish an entirely new meteorological theory – that of the anticyclone. His book *Meteorographica* is still required reading at seats of meteorology.

He let none of his studies interfere with his travels, and in 1850 he set off to explore the Zambesi territory 'and examine the Hottentots'. The Hottentots resented being examined, but Galton so impressed their chief by riding into his kraal in full hunting pink, straddling an ox that 'snuffled like a war horse', that the native promised to stop killing the missionaries who had been annoying him.

Two years later he returned to England and compiled his famous *Art of Travel, or Shifts and Contrivances Available in Wild Countries*. The book is entirely composed of practical advice and hints and tips – all no doubt effective, but some distinctly messy: 'A raw egg broken into a boot before putting it on greatly softens the leather;' 'to bait lice that will otherwise infest your clothes, take half an ounce of mercury and mix it with old tea leaves reduced to a paste by mastication and salivation, roll the paste into little beads and hang them round the neck on a string;' 'treacle and limejuice spread on the gums will alleviate the looseness of the teeth caused by scurvy.'

Such oddities abound. But the book as a whole is a remarkable compendium. It covers the organising of an expedition; surveying the site for a camp; the construction of boats and rafts and huts and tents; the care of firearms, and the best way to fire them effectively (as, for instance, from the back of a galloping horse); clothes, food, and first-aid for the safari; distress signalling; fishing without a line; mountaineering; finding bearings; and The Management of Savages ('A frank, joking, but determined manner is the best'). Reading it, one feels that every instruction has been tried by Galton personally and not found wanting.

But *The Art of Travel*, long and detailed as it is, was by no means his only writing activity. Like many Victorians he felt that an idle moment was an instrument of the devil. He wrote for the British Association a solemn paper on the genetic reasons for the enormous backsides of Hottentot women, which he had measured from a properly modest distance with surveying instruments and translated into statistical terms by means of trigonometry and logarithms. Less solemnly, he compiled a *Beauty Map of Britain*, also based on his beloved statistics, showing that all the prettiest girls were in London. (Oddly, the map had its biggest sale in Aberdeen, where according to Galton the girls were least attractive.) His filing systems of statistics naturally revealed other oddments of information – most of it apparently useless – and by some curious deduction of his own the prevalence of colour-blindness in Quakers led him to a completely new method of classifying fingerprints, which Scotland Yard uses to this day. The increasing popularity of bicycling led him to invent the cyclometer for recording speed and mileage, and the goggles used by skin divers evolved from his luminous spectacles for 'deep-sea investigators'.

As he grew older (he lived to be 89) he attached himself fanatically to the study of eugenics (a word he coined). The tens of thousands of questionnaires he had acquired in his statistical investigations, divided and subdivided into innumerable categories, aided his investigation of the notion that the entire human race might be brought to absolute perfection by the selective breeding of the best people in it. He was devoted to his wife, Louisa, but the idea of love could not possibly have entered into his cold calculations. *Hereditary Genius* is concerned only with the matching of perfect physical, intellectual, and moral specimens. The Fellows of the Royal Society thought it a profoundly interesting idea; paters in their Victorian drawing-rooms discussed it with their families; Mechanics' Institutes throughout the country provided the book for their students; literary societies debated it; parsons based their sermons on it; bishops wrote to *The Times* about it. But no one seized on it as a practical possibility until, eleven years after Galton's death in 1911, that ignoble creature Heinrich

8 *Gerolamo Cardano*
odds and universal joints

IN HIS ROOM in the palace in Edinburgh, Archbishop Hamilton lay gasping for breath after one of the vicious seizures that afflicted him. The room was tightly closed and curtained, the heavy hangings of his great bed gave off faint clouds of dust as he clutched at them for support, and in the middle of the room a charcoal brazier smoked and raised the temperature of the room to a stifling degree. Even the young woman who had recently left the Archbishop's bed had found the room unbearably oppressive and considered her purse of money well earned as she made her way home through the damp streets of the city.

Her departure through a wicket door at the rear of the palace coincided with the less furtive arrival of the renowned Italian doctor, Gerolamo Cardano, at the main entrance. Besides being a distinguished medical practitioner, Cardano was a mathematician, metaphysician, astrologer, designer, inventor, and theologian. But his present task was the cure of a bodily ill. He had set out from Padua in September 1551 and the journey by horseback, coach, and galley had taken nine months. He made haste now to deal with his upper-crust patient, who had summoned him with the offer of 'all the riches of my revenue' if he could relieve his asthma.

The treatment Cardano prescribed, though it was considered magical in its success, was no more than common sense. The Archbishop's excesses in eating, drinking, and high living were changed to a spartan regimen. He was forbidden to 'toy with harlots before dinner,' ordered to open his bedroom

47

windows, and 'to ride daily upon the back of a gentle horse.'
The brazier was banished and he was bidden to take ten hours'
sleep each night after a supper of ass's milk, honey, and chicken
broth. Good stuff; and, not surprisingly, the Archbishop gained
much relief. In gratitude he begged Cardano to call on him 'in
any circumstances that give you trouble.'

Cardano's life was one long trouble. Born in 1501, he was the
bastard son of Fazio Cardano, a feckless mathematician and
lawyer who might have been wealthy if Gerolamo's mother
hadn't had a parasitic family who continually milked Fazio's
coffers while he was engaged in learned pursuits.

Gerolamo too was feckless. But his fecklessness was turned to
good use. Gambling away many of his leisure hours while a
medical student at Padua university he calculated the chances
of throwing a particular number in a game of dice: 'Events may
be of three kinds: the impossible (as it might be the throwing of
a 7 with a single die), the certain (as the certainty that one side
of a thrown die must fall uppermost), and the probable (as it
might be that a 6 should fall uppermost at the first throw of the
die). If the impossible is set down as 0 and the certain as 1, then
all the degrees of probability in between may be calculated in
fractions.' Thus the chances of a particular side of a die falling
uppermost are $\frac{1}{6}$. This is the first Law of Probability, and every
gambler nowadays knows it. But it was Cardano who first
worked it out.

He also achieved many 'firsts' in his wide studies outside
medicine. In the matter of inventions he was a minor Leonardo.
He invented the universal joint that is used in the transmission
shaft (the Cardan-shaft, as it's widely known) of every motor-
car; he worked out the design of the first combination lock (it
would open only when certain cogs were aligned in an order
predetermined by a series of words or numerals); he devised a
system of numerical shorthand that was much used by algebraists in the public debates that were a popular form of amusement during the Renaissance; and he wrote countless books
that were best-sellers of their time (one of them, *The Practice of
Arithmetic*, sold many thousands of copies and brought him a

fortune in golden crowns).

Apart from such practical matters he also made notable contributions to the pseudo-sciences of astrology, geomancy, graphology, and palmistry; and delved deep into theology, and, of course, medicine.

Skilled though he was in medicine, he was granted his degree only after coming before the Faculty three times for election. 'No doubt,' he records, 'the disgrace attaching to my bastardy, the odium of my attendance in places where dice and cards were the idols, and my rudeness in dispute, were more than the sages of the Faculty could digest.' At last, however, at the end of the semester in autumn 1525, the court usher banged his staff three times on the ground and announced:

'Gerolamo Cardano, laureate in medicine, you are now by your learning qualified to sit among the princes of the earth. Go, and heal those who need you.'

The princes of the earth, however, were by no means keen to have him among them. In Milan they even barred him from practising by refusing to admit him to the Faculty of Medicine. His methods were too unorthodox. He had no bedside manner; he scorned placebos; and too often told rich patients that their stomach pains were caused by eating too much, and their pudendal infections by copulating too promiscuously – both of which statements were invariably true.

One of the few to whom his bluntness of speech was acceptable was Pope Paul III, who had approved one of Cardano's many astrological treatises, a *Life of Christ* in horoscope form, and now invited him to enter the papal service as astrologer and physician. The appointment brought him much prestige; it also made him many enemies, including the great algebraists of the day Tartaglia and Scaliger, both of whom Cardano had defeated in public debate and who now had the worm of envy burrowing into them.

It was through Pope Paul that Cardano gained many noble patients, including the asthmatic Archbishop Hamilton. But when he returned from Edinburgh in January 1553 the plots wrought by his enemies were thickening. His great pleasure was to see his children again. He had two sons, Giovanni and Aldo, and a daughter, Chiara. None of them was worthy of much joy. Chiara was a whore, Giovanni later became a murderer (he killed his wife by baking her a poisoned cake), and Aldo was to become public torturer under the Inquisition. These proclivities, however, Cardano failed to see through the mists of his extravagant affection. He also failed to see that they were ganging up with his rivals to bring about his downfall.

It was a simple enough task even without recourse to the accusation of heresy – the most dreaded word in Renaissance Italy. He had too often challenged – rudely and in public – the efficacy of the treatments, diagnoses, and prognoses meted out by his fellow doctors gathered round the bed of some rich patient. His recommendation of fresh air and gentle exercise had too often proved successful in mild ailments; and he had once achieved the unbelievable by curing a woman of tuberculosis through merely sending her to live in the mountains of Switzerland. His successes were said to be the results of quackery or because he was in league with the dark powers. Evidence was easily accumulated by his children from the voluminous writings in his studio, many of which pointed to his study of the *Malleus Maleficarum*, the fifteenth-century book on witchcraft which was forbidden reading in the medical profession.

Gradually Cardano found himself faced by an implacable wall of rejection. He could secure no professorship in any of the colleges and his patients dwindled to a handful. Reduced to poverty, his mind frayed a little and he wandered the streets in strange garb, shouting impieties and imprecations. The imprecations were understandable; the impieties too for that matter; but, with the network of the Inquisition flourishing in city, village, and vineyard, a shadowy hand could be kept on any citizen; shadowy records were accumulated as they were later to be in Nazi Germany. It was not good to shout impieties.

Chiara, his daughter, died of general paralysis of the insane caused by syphilis; but Giovanni and Aldo continued to weave their schemes against him, rewarded by the Inquisition for every scrap of information, true or false, they could contribute to the records against their father.

At last the dossier was complete. On 13 October 1570 Cardano was arrested in Bologna on the orders of the new Pope, Pius V, whose views on the casting of horoscopes of Christ were very different from those of Paul III. The ageing doctor (he was now sixty-nine) was accused of 'supreme blasphemies' and 'monstrous heresies' and of 'caring for his patients' bodies at the expense of their souls.' (This last was because on his own admission he had often ignored the papal bull directing that no doctor should treat any patient who had not made a full confession of his sins.)

He was flung into jail and allowed to languish for eleven weeks before being brought to trial. Then he was returned to jail and left uncertain as to his fate – that being a torture in itself. But he managed to recall mistily through his ravaged mind Hamilton's promise to help 'in any circumstances that give you trouble.' He wrote at once, smuggling the letter out by a jailer whose wife he had once cured of 'a monstrous flux'. It took many months for a reply to arrive; but at last the Archbishop sent word by special emissary to Rome that Cardano deserved the benefit of any doubts that could be cast upon his heretical deviations – 'For he is a scholar who troubles only with preserving and curing the bodies in which God's souls may live to their greatest length.'

Hamilton's plea was successful. Cardano was released and was once again to be seen in the streets, no longer shouting oaths and impieties but making endless notes on scraps of paper as he sought for patients among the destitute, to whom he devoted the rest of his life.

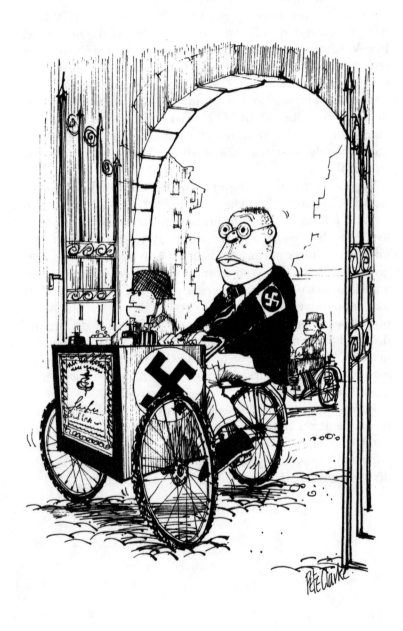

9 *Theodore Morell the Führer's tricycling quack*

ONE DAY in 1936 'Professor' Theodore Morell received a summons that was to change the course of his own and a good many other lives: he was commanded to report to the Chancellery in Berlin to consult with Hitler's doctors about an 'eczema' of the Führer's right leg.

At that time Morell was sixty-four and had a curious but flourishing practice in Berlin which was listed as a 'clinic for intimate diseases'. Medical reference books revealed little about him except that he was born in Hamburg in 1872 and had graduated from Leipzig with the minimum qualifying degree in 1900.

But however small the degree the certificate accompanying it was an impressive scroll of parchment complete with seal. Intended to decorate the young Bachelor of Medicine's consulting-room wall, Morell saw a much better use for it. He fixed the framed certificate on the front of a box tricycle and pedalled from town to town on market days, holding 'consultations' in an easily erected booth beside the tricycle, which contained a veritable pharmacy of drugs, placebos, unguents, and surgical instruments.

Market-square quackery was hardly ethical, but it was extremely profitable – particularly as he adopted the dress and speech of a learned professor: ill-fitting and stained clothes, velvet Wagnerian beret, flowing tie, and an incomprehensible patter that blinded his listeners with science and struck both terror and relief into their hearts: 'The trachea extends vertically from the larynx downward, bifurcating to form the bronchi, and is reinforced by cartilaginous rings lined with membrane with an epithelium composed of columnar cells.'

He would then go on to explain that, should the trachea become clogged with dust or anything, death would result, but that a perfect safeguard would be found in his patented 'filter' pills that at all times ensured the dissolution of anything tending to obstruct the windpipe. Having sold innumerable boxes of pills he would invite hypochondriac patients for private consultations about their individual complaints.

By sycophantically listening to their tales of woe and treating them with heavy doses of narcotics and stimulants, Morell made a lot of money, and a reputation as a 'character'. He was photographed with his portable consulting-room by Heinrich Hoffmann, who in 1922 became Hitler's official photographer, and the picture appeared in the German equivalent of *The Tatler*. Now, top Berliners beat a path to Morell's door – or, rather, to his booth, which he continued to use, just as he continued to use his odd vehicle for 'house visits'. Even when Hitler summoned him to the Chancellery that day in 1936 he insisted on pedalling there on his tricycle, though he was accompanied by motor-cycle outriders of the S.S. *Leibstandarte*.

Doctors Walter Conti, Siegfried Giesing, and Ernst Brandt, who were part of the Führer's large medical entourage, described Morell as 'fat and grubby, cringing in manner, and with small pig-like eyes that glittered with greed behind thick pebble glasses.' Notwithstanding these unpleasing characteristics Hitler at once accepted 'the Professor', as he called him – Morell being quick to take advantage of his new but unwarranted title. There sprang up between them a relationship not unlike that between a medieval king and his jester. There was mutual suspicion, and mutual trust too; the trust on Hitler's part grew into a dependence he resented but which Morell could use as a form of blackmail.

According to Hitler's valet, Heinze Linge, who was present and helped Hitler undress at that first examination in 1936, the basis of the blackmail was established almost at once. Morell's

examination of the sores on the Führer's leg led him to suspect
that they were the lesions of syphilis in its secondary stage. No
doubt the other doctors had come to the same conclusion, but
deemed it wise to keep it to themselves. Morell, however, had
no such inhibitions. He wrested from Hitler the fact that in
1910, when he was living the life of an impoverished roustabout
in Vienna, he had had a liaison with a Jewish whore; he had
received no treatment for the consequent syphilitic rash and
sores, which subsequently cleared up – as is normal in the primary stage of the disease. 'The illness', Morell mumbled while
soapily rubbing his hands together, 'does not necessarily pass
with the visible signs! Rarely in fact. The microbe *Spirochaeta
pallida* goes on destroying the tissues unsuspected for years and
eventually its successful ravages reveal themselves in such
symptoms as this supposed eczema. But I can cure you, my
Führer – though I should need to be in constant attendance
upon you.'

There was no difficulty about that. Hitler, who was a para-
gon of hypochondria, suffered from insomnia and flatulence,
and was neurotic about growing fat, becoming impotent, and
smelling of his own sweat. His coterie of doctors had tried to
jolly him into forgetting such trivia, but had been threatened
with dismissal in consequence. Morell crept to his aid with
cringing sympathy and 'anti-gas' pills containing strychnine
and atropine, with injections of an extract of bulls' testicles in
grape sugar, and with massive doses of dextrine, pervatin, caf-
feine, cocaine, prozymen, ultraseptyl, and vitamins. It became
Linge's job to ensure that at every meal the proper tablets were
taken in the right order and that Morell was always on hand
with his hypodermic when injections were due.

Having possessed himself of the Führer's guilty secret and his
resentful trust, Morell built with them an impregnable reputation. Doctors Giesing and Brandt attacked him for stuffing
the Führer with poisonous substances: the result was Giesing's
dismissal and Brandt's despatch to a concentration camp.
Their colleagues understandably held their tongues. Morell
then feathered his own nest by blatantly advertising his patent

medicines as 'under the Führer's patronage', for which he was
rewarded with large orders from the armed forces and numerous requests to treat private patients. Gestapo records discovered after the war showed that he had salted away a
millionaire's fortune from these sidelines, though his appointment to Hitler's medical entourage was an honorary one.

He never discarded his 'character' part. Though he was not
permitted to be beyond Hitler's call, his tricycle (refurbished
with the Nazi eagle and swastika painted on its sides) was
equipped with two-way radio; Morell was to be seen tricycling
through the bombed streets of whatever town harboured the
Führer, answering desperate calls from rich top-ranking Nazis
who wanted to avail themselves of his services. His untidiness
and grubbiness increased. The historian Trevor-Roper described him as 'a gross but deflated old man of cringing man-
ners, inarticulate speech, and the hygienic habits of a pig.' But
he is important to world history, because he did cure the
Führer's 'eczema'.

The cure, for what it was worth, had been effected by injections of Salvarsan, an antibiotic discovered after 606 experiments by the German physiologist Paul Ehrlich in 1910. But
much deeper damage than was manifested by sores on the leg
had been done: the microbe *Spirochaeta pallida* had attacked the
lower centres of Hitler's brain and the result was a slow de-
generation that was beyond arrest. It became steadily worse as
the war progressed. Field-Marshal Heinz Guderian, writing in
1951, said:

'The external evidence of his illness became increasingly apparent . . . not only his left hand but the entire left side of his
body shook. In sitting he had to hold his right hand over his left,
his right leg crossed over his left in order to make the constant
shaking less noticeable. His gait became shuffling, and his pos-
ture bent . . . he had to have a chair placed under him when he
wanted to seat himself.'

It was convenient for Morell that the symptoms of
Parkinson's disease are similar. He was able to keep Hitler's
secret and at the same time explain the palsy. Naturally, no

hint was ever published that the Führer was not in perfect health. But the price he had to pay was to be stuffed with the poisons Morell continually administered to comfort him in his hypochondriacal illnesses. After the attempted assassination in July 1944, twenty-eight different pills were found scattered around the floor, and all had come from the Führer's bomb-torn clothes. They were his daily supply, and his first thoughts were for their recovery so that he could get through the rest of the day without missing any of his doses. Like a drug pedlar, Morell had made certain that his patient had become addicted.

The Führer remained in his comforter's power till a week before his suicide in the Chancellery bunker on 30 April 1945. On 24 April, having made the decision to end the Third Reich with his own death, Hitler ordered a number of his entourage including Morell (and, incidentally, Hermann Göring, who was another drug addict supplied by the 'Professor') to leave the Berlin battle zone and seek safety in the south, where the tattered remains of the German army fought toward Berlin in a hopeless attempt to drive the Russians from the capital. But there was no safety. Morell was arrested by American troops and died shortly afterward of a cerebral haemorrhage.

It is a moot point whether Morell prolonged or shortened Hitler's life with his attentions. What is certain is that for nine years the megalomaniac leader of the Third Reich was in the power of a quack doctor who had ranted in market places and made a fortune out of the gullible.

10 *Peter Roget*
snap! crackle!! pop!!!

'IT IS NOW my pleasure to introduce our Guest of Honour – one of the most remarkable men it has been my lot to encounter; who is remarkable not only for his sprightliness at a considerable age but also for the width of his vision and the scope of his activities; a man who varies from the conventional mould to a marked degree. Gentlemen: Doctor Peter Roget.'

The speaker was George Augustus Sala, ace reporter of the *Daily Telegraph*; the occasion a dinner at Sala's club in Covent Garden in 1859 to honour not only Dr Roget but also the success of his *Thesaurus of English Words and Phrases, classified and arranged so as to facilitate the Expression of Ideas and assist in Literary Composition*, which had been published seven years earlier and had achieved a remarkable success.

The Thesaurus, a compendium of words arranged under different sub-divisions of six primary classes – Abstract Relations, Space, Material World, Intellect, Volition, and Sentient and Moral Powers – was intended to help those searching to express themselves within those classified ideas. It was in fact a vast book of synonyms arranged with the orderly precision that had typified Roget's life.

Though a Londoner by birth – he was born in Soho – Roget had no English blood in his veins, which in a way makes his *magnum opus* the more remarkable. His parents were Huguenots who had fled France, and Peter was born in 1779, when his father was Pastor of the French Protestant Church in Threadneedle Street. His work on the Thesaurus was not begun until he was seventy-one and was, to him, more of an occupation for leisure hours than a task of formidable magnitude – which is what it would have seemed to anyone else. He had to list thousands upon thousands of words, and set them down in opposing columns that offered both synonyms and antonyms respecting the same basic idea; it might well have formed the life work of a lesser man. Roget completed it in only four years – though admitting in his preface that he had had the idea half a century earlier and had assembled the beginnings of 'a classed catalogue of words' and had often contemplated 'its extension and improvement'.

The methodical precision with which Roget's life was to be ordered could have been remarked by his progress at his first school – a private one directed by a Mr Chauvet in Kensington – where he showed a remarkable aptitude for mathematics, which science he found 'remarkably easy to comprehend because of its systematic nature.' From London he moved with his mother, now widowed, and sister Suzanne to Edinburgh. That was in 1793. Two years later, at the age of sixteen, he entered the University to study medicine – which he also found organised so systematically that he had no difficulty in qualifying M.D. (with honours and a gold medal thrown in for his researches into Pulmonary Consumption) in three years and getting recorded as 'the most outstanding graduate of the year 1798'.

Those researches were conducted by what were then considered the most unorthodox methods. In Edinburgh Infirmary he walked the wards, contracted typhus and was written off as beyond recovery, only to puzzle the medicos by recovering completely in a fortnight. To widen his scope, he boldly called a conference of doctors from all over England. It was the first medical conference ever to be held, and Edinburgh University footed the bill. Its purpose was to pool all available knowledge of Pulmonary Consumption, and the visiting doctors could scarcely believe that not only were they being addressed by a student of eighteen, but that he had organised the conference with a high degree of efficiency and that he recorded all their

contributions to the discussion in a shorthand of his own inven-
tion. (It approximated to today's Speedwriting.)

He anticipated Samuel Smiles by living by, if not actually
originating, the maxim 'A place for everything, and everything
in its place.' His boundless curiosity challenged the memory,
but its fruits were filtered through innumerable card index
systems and files arranged, as his Thesaurus was to be, under
subjects and sub-subjects. For that reason – plus, of course, the
extraordinary percipience of his mind – he could range widely
in his studies and activities, yet keep every hour orderly, every
scrap of information systematically stored.

Practically the only upset in Roget's early life was his arrest
in Geneva in 1803. He was there tutoring two boys, the children
of a wealthy Manchester man, and on the shattering of the
Peace of Amiens by Napoleon was threatened with internment
as an Englishman. He was quickly able to prove however, that
his father was a citizen of Geneva and that he himself was as
French as the blood in his veins; whereupon he was released
and returned to England via Frankfurt with his charges – ruf-
fled by the perfidy of France but otherwise unharmed.

He was still only twenty-four, but he quickly terminated a
spell as private physician to the Marquess of Lansdowne's son
('a sinecure of idlenesse') and went off to found a medical
school in Manchester, to plan a five-year series of weekly two-
hour lectures on physiology to be given to the Manchester
Literary and Philosophical Society, and to take on sec-
retaryships and presidencies of many diverse organisations.
This dynamo of a man coped easily with all these activities
without in anyway neglecting a thriving medical practice. One
would have thought his days were pretty well occupied.

By no means: he found life in the north lacking opportunities
'to stretch the mind' and moved to London in 1808. There he
found ample openings for his boundless energy. He took up an
appointment as physician to the Spanish Embassy, re-estab-
lished a busy medical practice of his own, became one of the
founders of the Northern Dispensary and the Medical and Chi-
rurgical Society of London, delivered lectures at the Russell

Scientific and Literary Institution, and was a co-founder of London University and chairman of its Faculty of Medicine. The Prime Minister, Lord Liverpool, commissioned him and the social reformer Jeremy Bentham to report on London's sewage system; the Royal College of Physicians asked him to undertake an investigation into the medical treatment of convicts in Millbank Prison; and the Theatre of Anatomy in Great Windmill Street appointed him its principal examiner.

As if these demanding occupations were not enough, treatises, contributions to learned and popular journals, and books poured from his pen. He contributed thirty-one articles to the *Encyclopaedia Britannica* and became compiler, editor and publisher of the *Cyclopaedia of Popular Medicine*, which offered to a general readership the elucidation of matters that had hitherto been considered sacredly esoteric. He also found time to get married in 1824 at the age of forty-five and sire two children before his wife, possibly unable to keep up with the pace of his exuberant existence, died in 1831.

Evidently there was also space in his polymerous mind for what he called 'lighthearted recreations'. He devised a chess formula for moving a Knight from any specified square to any specified square of the other colour traversing every square on the board but repeating none. This led him to invent the pocket chess-board used today and to a request from the *Illustrated London News* to pose a chess problem for the amusement of their readers each week. (Thus he became one of the earliest chess correspondents.) More importantly, he invented a logologarithmic machine in the form of a slide rule graduated to be a measure of the powers of numbers; and for this he was elected a Fellow of the Royal Society. As if membership of that august body were not enough he took on the post of Secretary in 1827 and held it until he was seventy. His other 'inventive experiments', as he called them, included a calculating machine and a balance unaffected by friction.

Since his entire life had been concerned with the acquisition of knowledge it was in no way surprising that he should want to disseminate that knowledge to the widest possible audience.

'The Societies of my acquaintance', he wrote to his uncle, Sir Samuel Romilly, 'are Very Fine and of inestimable value, but to address them is to me often like preaching to the Converted. It is of greater moment to me that a wider congregation should be able to share with me the mighty works of the Creator, which extend throughout the boundless regions of space, and whose comprehensive plans embrace Eternity.' His way of engaging that wider congregation was, characteristically, to form a Society for the Diffusion of Useful Knowledge, and to start off its library by turning out a whole series of manuals, somewhat similar to today's 'part-works,' on an immense variety of subjects. One of the manuals was a potted and popularised version of a lecture he had given to the Royal Institution on the possibility of electromagnetic galvanism becoming 'a likely substitute for candles'.

Sala, it must now be clear, was in no way exaggerating when he introduced Roget as 'remarkable'. He lived to be ninety and never stopped working, suffered no diminution of his faculties except that of hearing, and was interested to the last in all that went on 'in honor of the Power, Wisdom, and Goodness of God'. Since he was the least egotistic of men he would not have been troubled to foresee that posterity would forget him completely except for his remarkable Thesaurus. All word users are in his debt: not least, the advertisement copywriter who, searching for a slogan for Rice Krispies, found the very thing he wanted in Section 402 of the Thesaurus under the heading 'Sudden and Violent Noise': *Snap . . . crackle . . . pop.*

Immortality indeed.

MOWBRAYS ECCENTRIC SERIES

Other titles in preparation

Eccentric Soldiers	by Carol Kennedy
Eccentric Doctors	by Alan Wykes
Eccentric Clerics	by John Lastingham
Eccentric Explorers	by Ann Novotny
Eccentric Collectors	by Carol Kennedy
Eccentric Golfers	by George Houghton
Eccentric Scientists	by Dick Dempewolff
Eccentric Boxers	by John Cottrell
Eccentric Sailors	by Carol Kennedy
Eccentric Musicians	by Alan Wykes
Eccentrics of the Gun	by J. A. Maxtone Graham